Raw Food Diet

A Quick Simple Guide to Help You Lose Weight, Look Younger and Boost Health More Effectively

Sarah Sparrow

PUBLISHED BY:
Sarah Sparrow

Disclaimer

The information contained in this book is for general information purposes only. The information is provided by the authors and while we endeavor to keep the information up to date and correct, we make no representations or warranties of any kind, express or implied, about the completeness, accuracy, reliability, suitability or availability with respect to the book or the information, products, services, or related graphics contained in the book for any purpose. Any reliance you place on such information is therefore strictly at your own risk.

TABLE OF CONTENTS

Introduction

There are several books about raw food dieting, but none quite like this one. Here you'll find practical, useful, down-to-earth advice from leading doctors, practitioners, and raw food experts. You'll discover these tips are easy to follow. Their explanations are straightforward – free from industry jargon. Their advice is as specific as it can be (though, of course, how you take it up is up to you).

Whether they're suggesting how to sprout seeds and nuts, how to alkalize your body, or how to reverse aging and disease, theirs are words to the wise. We already know much about our bodies and how they work; now we can take that information and pursue optimal health.

There have been significant breakthroughs in understanding the benefits of raw food dieting in the past few years. We are equipped with more information which allows us to make better decisions about our health and longevity. We also have more choices in how to obtain the fresh, organic food we need – choices such as where to shop and how to buy, how to grow our own food, the pluses and minuses of fasting – even which questions to ask our doctors before we begin.

Where do you find the answers? You can ask your doctor, of course – but does that doctor really have the time to answer all of your questions, or do they even recommend a healthy diet in addition to your host of medications? You can look things up online, but this is time consuming and can lead to confusion and conflicting information. And you can always ask your friend and family – but are their solutions appropriate for you?

Be assured, you're not the only person with these questions. Others share your concerns – and yes, even some of your doubts and confusion about what's best for you and what you should be doing to protect your health at this time in your life. With so many concerns in common, it only made sense for us to ask experts the questions you have – and then bring those answers together in one common place that we all can share.

This book is that place. So if there's something you've been wondering about a raw food diet, just ask. Chances are very good that you'll find the answers here.

Turn to the Contents and you'll quickly see that this is more than an introduction to raw food dieting. Yes, this book discusses all the aspects of a raw food diet, but it also tells you what can go wrong and how to prevent it from happening. This is more than a book about raw food it's a book that puts you in charge of your health.

Chapter 1: WHY GO RAW?

What is the Raw Food Diet?

A raw food diet consists primarily of fruits, vegetables, nuts, sprouts, and beans, in their most natural, or raw, state. The raw food craze which seems to be sweeping the nation isn't a new or novel idea by any stretch, but it is certainly gaining a wider range of acceptance now that raw food restaurants are cropping up all over the country.

To truly understand the benefit of a raw food diet is to accept that it's not a diet at all, it's a lifestyle focused on health and wellness. Weight loss is a side effect experienced by many practitioners, but even better than the shedding of unwanted pounds is the drastic reduction of chronic pain and illness.

Diabetes, heart disease, asthma, and other chronic illnesses that are responsible for millions of deaths annually, are controlled, even cured completely, as a result of following a raw food diet.

How Hard Is It to Switch to a Diet of Raw Food?

Switching to a raw food diet takes very little effort and is actually quite easy! Whether your goal is to go 70% raw, 100% raw, or somewhere in between, making the switch isn't difficult at all once you've set your mind to it.

For some it takes a major health crisis to find the inspiration to take their health seriously, for others they just need to witness the dramatic health improvement in a loved one to see the logic in making the switch for themselves.

Once you make the decision to go raw it's as easy as gathering ingredients from the produce section of your local grocery. Organic fruits and vegetables are the ideal ingredients to look for, as well as anything that hasn't been treated with heavy amounts of pesticides. Always wash your produce before consuming to ensure it's free of dirt, insects, or waxy coating.

Why You Will Love the Raw Food Diet

Once your body is free from the toxins of a diet rich in animal protein and processed foods, you'll be amazed at the boundless energy you experience each day.

Rare and chronic conditions can be permanently reduced, even cured, when consuming a diet of raw foods. The list of chronic illnesses and conditions which are drastically alleviated as a result of following a diet of raw foods is staggering enough to be influential in its own right.

Depression, hangovers, colds, menstrual cramps, headaches, varicose veins, diabetes, asthma, peptic ulcers, hypertension, constipation, arthritis - best yet, all of these can be dramatically improved with a blend of fruits and vegetables in the form of juice. Not only good for you, they taste great too!

Making the Transition to a Raw Food Diet Easy

Some people need to make drastic changes; others need to ease into change by incorporating small steps little by little. No matter which type of person you are, making the transition to a raw food diet is really quite simple.

You can start small by eliminating a serving of animal-based protein each day, replacing it with a fresh fruit or vegetable. Using this method, by the end of the week, you've eliminated a significant amount of unhealthy protein and have replaced it with a healthy, delicious form of protein which tastes great, and is great for you.

Following this same procedure, and taking small steps towards incorporating 70% or more raw food into your diet, you won't even miss the processed food and animal protein.

If you really want to reboot your system, eliminating processed food and animal-based protein quickly, then a juice fast is the fastest and easiest way to make the transition into a raw food diet. Simply create delicious, nutrient-rich drinks from fruits and vegetables purchased at your local grocery, whole food coop, or farmer's market.

Fruits and vegetables in their raw form are packed with micronutrients which fight disease, restore cell health, and reduce toxins in the body. The first few days may be a little difficult as your body purges years of built up toxins, and once the fog of carbohydrate addiction begins to lift your desire for processed food and animal-based protein will be a thing of the past.

Chapter 2: RAW BASICS

Starting a Raw Food Diet

Starting a raw food diet is only as difficult as you make it. If you go into dreading all of the sugary indulgences that you're giving up, you can be certain your healthy new lifestyle won't last very long. Consider how much better you'll feel when you're eating the diet your body was designed for!

Some choose to start slow, adding a serving of fruits and vegetables each day while slowly removing cooked food from their diet. Still others choose the extreme, cold turkey route and give up cooked food completely with a 10 day juice fast to reboot their system.

Maybe 10 days seems too long, so shoot for a week instead.

The important thing is that you try to do a little something each day, making sure to not beat yourself up if things aren't progressing at rapid pace. After all, it probably took you several years to reach a point where a raw food diet seems truly logical, old habits die hard. This is why it's so important to surround yourself with supportive, like-minded people who will help make the transition easier, especially when the dreaded food cravings occur.

Shopping for Raw Foods

The easiest way to avoid food cravings is to keep your kitchen well stocked with plenty of raw food options. Check the weekly advertisements for your local grocery to take advantage of special offers on fresh produce, preferably organic if you can find it.

Farmer's markets are another great way to get freshly picked, seasonal fruits and vegetables for a fraction of the price. Some grocery chains, like Whole Foods, have entire sections devoted to raw food, even going so far as stocking prepared raw food already packaged for convenience.

Something important to remember is that you are empowered! Even if your neighborhood grocer doesn't stock a wide selection of organic produce, ask them to order fruits and vegetables on your behalf. Tell them you want to buy in bulk, and then ask if they're willing to provide a discount for buying direct. Because you intend to be a regular customer in this manner, and they don't want to lose your business to competitor, many grocers will be more than happy to accommodate your needs. Other customers may also appreciate the introduction of organic options as well.

Regardless of where you choose to purchase your raw food, select those fruits and vegetables that you'll actually want to eat. There's plenty of time for experimenting with exotic foods and complicated recipes. The important thing right now is that you stock your kitchen with raw food and nothing but raw food, so when those detox cravings set in you'll have plenty of nutritious and delicious options to keep you feeling satisfied.

Tips on How to Store Raw Foods Properly

When purchasing bulk produce, make sure to buy it in various degrees of ripeness. Staggering your produce this way will ensure you've always got something ripe on hand without risking too much loss. Keep the cardboard boxes that your fruit is packaged in; this will allow for easy stacking, this will also drastically reduce uneven ripening and crushed produce.

Next, invest in an inexpensive shelving unit to place within a cool, dark closet. Produce is best stored at a room temperature, or slightly below, away from direct sunlight. Arrange your boxes of fruit with the ripest at the top of the shelf, and the least ripe at the bottom. Because you'll be using this as a pantry of sorts you will always be aware of what is ready to eat, and what will be ready to eat in the near future.

Should any of your produce go bad before you have a chance to enjoy it, don't worry! Simply add the fruits and vegetables to your compost pile. The worms in your soil will certainly appreciate the boost in nutrients, and your garden will thank you too.

How to Equip Your Kitchen for a Raw Food Diet

There's really only four key pieces of equipment you'll want to invest in for your new raw food kitchen, a juicer, a blender, a food processor and a dehydrator. Drinking juice blended from fresh fruits and vegetables is by far the easiest way to consume the proper amount of calories your body needs each day, which is why a juicer is the number one piece of equipment to purchase.

Smoothies are delicious, and like juicing it's a fantastic way to deliver nutrient food to your system quick and easily. The really nice thing about juices and smoothies is your body doesn't have to work so hard to process your food, allowing you to notice the benefits much sooner. Blenders can easily whip up smoothies in a matter of seconds, but they're also useful for making cold soups, spreads and nut butters, allowing you a wider range of options in your raw food diet.

Food processors are ideal for making sauces, puddings and spreads. Every bit as quick and effective as a blender, foods prepared in a food processor will retain some of their texture. Marinara sauce, pesto, anything you can imagine, simply add the ingredients to the food processor and chop away. You can also use your food processor to shred vegetables for your salad or raw pasta dishes.

Last is the dehydrator and definitely something on the advanced end of the spectrum for raw food dieters. Dehydrated fruits are delicious and easy to tote along for the busy raw foodist on the go. Dehydrated tomatoes have a higher lycopene content than raw tomatoes, which effectively demonstrates the importance of a dehydrator as a necessary piece of equipment for the serious raw foodist.

Why Consider the Source of Your Food?

The only difference between a regular banana and an organic banana is the price, right? Wrong.

Organic produce is better for a number of reasons, not the least of which is the lack of pesticides used during cultivation. Pesticides aren't just harmful to the pests that enjoy fresh produce; it's also harmful to the people that consume that food, no matter how well you think you've washed it first. When you purchase organic food, you are also supporting the farmer that took the time to nurture that plant by hand, all the way through the growth cycle and beyond.

Concerns on the Raw Food Diet

If you are currently taking medications or are under a doctor's care, please consult your physician before beginning any diet, this includes a raw food diet. This will help establish a baseline for your doctor to measure progress, or deficiencies, as you continue with your new healthy lifestyle. Do not stop taking your prescription medications until your doctor advises you to do so.

One of the most common concerns on a raw food diet is consuming the proper amount of nutrients each day. Many people assume that a raw food diet consisting of whole, plant-based ingredients is dangerously void of valuable protein, but this isn't the case at all. The highest concentration of protein in any source in the world comes from spirulina, blue green spiral algae that fed some of the greatest civilizations on this earth.

One of the great things about these highly concentrated protein sources is when they're raw they're easily absorbed. You get everything, you get all the protein, and you're not missing some of the amino acids that are degraded by heat. If you're not quite ready to eat an alga, that's okay, vegetables in general are good sources of protein, not in the same concentration as spirulina, but it's the same basic building blocks.

Some individuals experience a drop in their iron levels when starting a raw food diet, becoming borderline anemic as a result. An easy way to correct this is by consuming more leafy greens such as parsley, dandelion and spinach. Some of the summer fruits, like cherries, are very high in iron. Really the color gives it away, that bright red color of cherries indicates high iron content. There are also supplemental vitamins you can take during this transition which will give you the additional nutrients you need to get through without feeling depleted.

How to Save Money on a Raw Food Diet

Quite simply the easiest way to save money on a raw food diet is to grow your own. If that's not an option in your area, consider joining an organic farmer's cooperative. Or start a cooperative of your own; you only need five or six other people to get on board with you to start a movement within your community if one doesn't already exist.

Short of that, visit your local farmer's markets, buy in bulk, and take advantage of sales at your local grocery. Fruit really does grow on trees, if you have fruit trees in your neighborhood ask your neighbors if they're willing to share.

Common Mistakes on Raw Food Diet

Believe it or not, the most common mistake on a raw food diet is overeating. The general rule is to eat when you're hungry, but many of us eat to reduce stress, soothe emotions, be social, or any number of other reasons aside from actual hunger. Popping food into your mouth every time you think you might be hungry is no good on any diet, even a diet consisting of raw foods.

Another common mistake is trail mix. On the surface it would seem the perfect go-to snack for raw foodists, but this combination of nuts, dried fruits, sugar and salt is actually more difficult for your body to process compared to eating a small handful of nuts for breakfast, followed by a handful of dehydrated dates a little later.

Failure to consume enough leafy greens tends to affect nearly everyone starting a raw food diet. This is a concern because those leafy greens are such an amazing source of B vitamins such as folate. To avoid an iron deficiency, make sure your juice drinks contain a substantial amount of kale.

When stocking up on food for your raw food diet, be sure to reach for organic and locally grown varieties. Many people experience a detox effect a few days when starting a raw food diet and these challenging side effects are exacerbated by non-organic food that has been treated with pesticides. To make the transition smoother, reach for locally grown, organic produce.

Not getting enough sleep, or exercise, is another mistake common to individuals new to the raw food diet. Sleeping is important for your body's ability to heal itself and recovery. Just as you're giving your body premium fuel so you can enjoy optimal health, you need to give yourself ample time to rest and recover as well. The same goes for exercise. You're going to feel a renewed sense of energy unlike any you've known before, expend this excess energy by doing something positive for your body by building up your cardio and strengthening your heart.

Besides Cooked Food, What Foods Should You Avoid?

Some fruits and vegetables simply cannot be consumed raw, and even dehydrated they fail to reach an optimal level of edibility. White potato, sweet potato and eggplant are much too tough in their raw state, and don't taste that great without first being cooked. Kidney beans, chickpeas, and soybeans contain toxins in their raw state which are removed during the process of cooking, which also degenerate their nutritive value. The best way to consume chickpeas raw is to let them sprout first. Rhubarb cannot be consumed raw, its toxicity and foul flavor are removed during cooking, along with its nutritive value.

In addition to avoiding fruits and vegetables which are difficult to consume in their raw state, it's important to avoid other items such as sugar, salt, wheat and alcohol as well. As you increase your intake of fruits you'll be consuming plenty of natural sugars to more than satisfy your sweet tooth. The same goes for salt, you simply won't need it because raw fruits and vegetables taste great naturally. Because you'll be avoiding baked goods, there's little reason to need wheat in any form.

Chapter 3: SUCCESFULLY RAW

Tips on How to Stay on a Raw Food Diet

Transitioning to a raw food diet takes some time, remember you've been eating processed food your whole life and it takes a while to break old habits. The goal is to remove processed and cooked foods from your diet. Do this little by little, or make a drastic change if you like, either way you should still take it one day at a time.

Start your day with a 16 ounce glass of water with lemon juice added. Usually about a half a lemon will do. Lemons are a great source of vitamin C and will help cleanse toxins from your liver. For breakfast, enjoy a fresh green smoothie made from the fruits and vegetables of your choice. A fruit smoothie is another excellent choice for breakfast. Consuming your fruits and vegetables in the form of a smoothie for breakfast is a fantastic way to supercharge your body with nutrients and antioxidants. You'll be amazed at your abundant energy as a result compared to eating a breakfast laden with fat and carbohydrates.

If you'd rather not start your day with a smoothie or a green power drink, then enjoy some fresh fruit. Eat as much as you like, or need, to satisfy your hunger. If you happen to feel hungry a little later, enjoy a snack of fresh fruit, carrot sticks, or a small handful of nuts. These simple snacks are easy to tote around with you, and they provide a satisfying crunch along with their sweet taste.

It's okay to enjoy a serving of lightly baked fish for dinner if you're just getting started with the transition to a raw food diet. Remember your goal is to remove heavy, fat-laden foods, and processed food from your diet. Keep your plate filled with as many fresh fruits and vegetables as you can as you slowly remove cooked and processed food from your list of meal options. If you're convinced that you cannot part with your steak and potatoes, choose smaller portions until you're comfortable eliminating these foods from your life.

Start weaning yourself from all manner of dairy products, breads, processed grains, pasta and red meats. Likewise, it's very important to eliminate all forms of junk food from your diet. Easier said than done, I know, that's because these foods are very addictive and easy to overdo. In addition to these foods to avoid, you'll also want to remove all processed sugars from your diet. You won't really miss this processed sugar once your begin consuming naturally sweet foods.

When transitioning to raw foods you will be consuming a lot of fiber from your fruits and vegetables, so make sure you're drinking plenty of water throughout. Take it one day at a time and remind yourself frequently that you're doing something positive for yourself. As you start to enjoy the benefits of a raw food diet it will be motivational in its own right, inspiring you to continue on this healthy new path.

Failure is not possible! Do not beat yourself up if you're not seeing successful results as quickly as you would like. Far too often we hold ourselves to unrealistic standards which only serve to derail our progress. Do what you can each day; even if it's a single smoothie for breakfast, the momentum will come in its own time. Be proud of yourself! Pat yourself on the back for making healthy decisions that will reward you for the rest of your life.

Stop weighing yourself! Why do you measure success by a number that's bound to fluctuate from one day to the next? Instead, pick a single day each month to be your weigh-in day, and then stay away from the scale for the remainder of the month. Measure your progress by how you feel, not what the number on the scale reflects. The positive results you're looking for will reveal themselves in time in the form of loose garments, clearer skin, better sleep, less pain, and an overall sense of well-being.

Balancing Your Raw Food Diet

The best way to ensure a balance diet when eating raw food is to eliminate the word "diet" from your vocabulary. Far too often we think of a diet as restrictive and calorie conscious, whereas a raw food lifestyle is completely the opposite. Eat as much as you want, don't assume you can get buy on a few bananas and an avocado each day, this leads to malnutrition.

Eat high quality food; this does cost a little extra money. Balance is easily obtained by consuming superfoods like spirulina, goji berries and hemp seeds. It's much more difficult to follow a raw food diet in a colder climate, or a location with long winters because much of the tropical fruits you need for proper nutrition is out of season half of the year. If you can't purchase fruits and vegetables in bulk for the purpose of ripening at home, consider starting a hydroponic growing system to ensure easy access to abundant, fresh produce all year round.

The most common imbalance noted among people who are new to a raw food diet is a deficiency in vitamins D, and B, as well as Iron. This is easily corrected by consuming the proper amount of dark, leafy green vegetables each day. Many assume a single salad is sufficient and this simply isn't the case. In truth you should be consuming at least a pound of leafy greens per day. The easiest way to ensure you're meeting the recommended daily allowance is by juicing. If you haven't yet purchased a juicer as part of your raw food kitchen, do so as quickly as possible.

Getting Enough Protein

A major point of contention between meat-eaters and raw foodists centers on the topic of protein. It's certainly true that one of the building blocks required by every cell in our body is protein, but that doesn't mean the best source of protein for your body comes from animals. Many cardiovascular problems can be traced back to consuming animal-based proteins, whereas it's been shown time and time again that plant-based proteins reverse the damage done by eating a red meat.

Protein is present in fruits, vegetables, and leafy greens. Getting enough protein is easily accomplished by eating plenty of raw produce each day. Eat a large salad each day packed with raw fruits, vegetables and nuts. Juicing is another great way to ensure you're getting plenty of plant-based protein each day. Don't deny yourself delicious, fresh foods, and experiment with plenty of variety to ensure you're getting plenty of nutrients. Raw sources of protein include:

- Nuts
- Seeds
- Avocado
- Sprouts
- Beans
- Sprouted grains
- Gobi berries
- Spiraling (blue green algae)
- Spinach
- Kale
- Broccoli

Sprouting is another way to ensure your diet is rich in a healthy source of protein. Sprouting is actually quite simple and rewarding. Nuts and seeds contain enzyme inhibitors, a toxic substance that protects the nuts and seed. Ingesting raw nuts and seeds in this manner can lead to irritation and digestive problems such as diverticulitis and irritable bowel syndrome. By soaking and sprouting your seeds and nuts you're effectively removing the enzyme inhibitors which also convert your food into a living food which is very beneficial to your health.

Getting Enough Iron

The mineral iron is necessary for oxygen transportation and cell growth. For most people, their primary source of iron and B-12 comes from animal products. As you make the transition to a raw food diet, eliminating red meat and animal products from your diet, a deficiency of iron is likely to occur. Make sure you're getting plenty of minerals in your diet by consuming food rich in mineral. Some of these include:

- Apples
- Oranges
- Bananas
- Grapes
- Peanuts
- Almonds
- Cashews
- Bok Choy
- Dandelion
- Spinach
- Leafy Greens

Nearly every person has removed dandelion from their front yard without realizing the many benefits of this hardy plant. Aside from being a potent source of iron and other minerals, dandelion also includes vitamins A, E, and C, as well as silica which is essential for healthy hair, skin and nails. Many people think of dandelion as a weed, but when you think of it a weed is simply a plant growing in the wrong place. Once you realize all the amazing health benefits of dandelion it's growing in exactly the right place. Dandelion is a bit bitter, so mix it in with a salad that also includes some drizzled orange juice and fresh raspberries.

Keeping It Interesting

Variety is vital when eating a raw food diet. There are so many fruits, vegetables, nuts, beans, and sprouts, as well as ways to prepare them. Being bored with the same meal night after a night should never be a problem. Raw food restaurants are cropping up all over the world, easily demonstrating how delicious and satisfying raw food meals can be.

Many people are won over to a raw food diet with smoothies, green drinks and desserts. Chocolate shakes, tortes and decadent treats are still possible with a creative balance of fruits, nuts and sweet ingredients. Experiment with ingredients and their preparation, you'll be amazed how easy it is to enjoy gourmet meals that are great for you.

Making the Raw Food Diet Work

The more simply you eat, the better your results, and the easiest way to do this is with breakfast. Enjoy a large morning meal of a large variety of fruits, or make a smoothie of your favorite fruit. Make it delicious and enjoyable, but eat enough to feel satisfied. If breakfast is all you can handle in the beginning, that's perfectly fine! Add fruits and vegetables with each meal, working up to a completely raw diet over time. This approach will not only allow your body time to adjust to benefits of a raw food diet, but your mind as well.

Few realize how addictive processed and cooked foods can be, and lifelong habits are hard to break. Adjustment is to be expected, and takes time. Nothing happens overnight, including the transition to a raw food diet. Try some low-fat, vegan, and savory recipes if you feel a complicated, complex meal is what your taste buds require. There are so many fabulous recipes available online and in raw food cookbooks, so don't be afraid to use your imagination when it comes to creating a diet that works for you.

Create a support group too. Even if your neighborhood isn't familiar with an organic, raw food lifestyle, you can raise awareness by starting a monthly potluck group. Gather regularly in a potluck fashion, sharing some of your favorite recipes while sampling the meals prepared by others. You'll be amazed at how easy it is to find inspiration and support as you focus on your new, healthy lifestyle.

How to Curb Cravings on a Raw Food Diet

Remember, this is a learning experience and a personal journey. Ups and downs are to be expected. Even if you dive right in and transition to a 100% raw diet then give in to a craving for a big juicy burger, don't beat yourself up. The important thing is you really focus on reducing the amount of processed foods and animal-based foods.

When you crave something sweet, reach for fruit. Listen to the needs of your body, and respond with the kind of food that's going to nourish your cells. Don't try to force yourself to eat something that doesn't appeal to you. Everyone has different tastes and needs. Instead, enjoy a broad variety of fruits, vegetables, nuts, seeds, sprouts and greens for the greatest amount of satisfaction.

How to Get Variety in a Raw Food Diet

A lack of variety is hardly a problem when enjoying a raw food diet. A lack of imagination, however, can lead to a lack of variety. When preparing a salad, include many different ingredients chopped and diced in a many different sizes, and shred a bit of your leafy greens as well, this will provide more texture to the salad. A fruit smoothie day after day can get monotonous, so change it up with green juices, sprouts and nuts.

One thing people miss when switching to a raw diet is the process of food preparation. For many the act of cooking a meal provides stress relief. There's no reason why you should deny yourself this simple pleasure when enjoying a raw food diet as well. Preparing nut butters, dehydrating food, and growing sprouts are all labor intensive, rewarding, and a fantastic way to add variety to your menu options.

How to Avoid the Dangers of a Raw Food Diet

The primary dietary concerns that go with the raw food diet center around deficiencies in iron, and B-12, but many don't realize that tooth decay can be a concern as well. Dental health tends to become an issue after several years of strict raw food consumption that doesn't include high enough levels of fatty acids and Omega 3, 6, and 9.

These deficiencies can easily be corrected with the addition of dietary supplements. However, supplements should be unnecessary if you're consuming superfoods such as:

- Hemp Seed
- Kelp
- Goji Berries
- Cacao
- Spirulina
- Maca
- Leafy Greens
- Wild Edibles

Superfoods are easily integrated into a raw food diet in the form of smoothies, juices, and other satisfying preparations.

Chapter 4: RAW BENEFITS

Cleanse with Raw Food Diet

When it comes to habits, they're not broken or made over night; the same is true for a raw food diet. To see if a raw food diet is suitable for you it's best to start with a cleanse. A cleanse is no different than following a raw food diet; it's simply a short-term commitment which allows you to obtain a baseline idea of what to expect as your body purges stored toxins.

Most raw food cleanses range from a short-term cleanse of 3-10 days, with 7 days as the goal for the majority of people undertaking a raw food challenge. To reverse years of damage from processed foods and animal products a longer cleanse of 30-60 days may be needed. If you're new to cleansing, start with three days to see how your body responds.

When undertaking a cleanse, choose a starting point when you won't be facing holiday meals, lunch meetings, or other interactions with cooked food. If you can, separate yourself from your normal environment. Spend a few weeks at the beach surrounded by plenty of fresh, raw food and a juicer for easy preparation. To ensure you're ready for a cleanse make sure you have plenty of fresh, organic fruits, vegetables and greens on hand so you always have a snack ready when cravings strike. A stocked pantry of flavor enhancers will ensure your food is never dull or boring, so make sure to have the following on hand before you begin your cleanse:

- Olive Oil - Cold Pressed
- Apple Cider Vinegar
- Honey - Raw
- Sea Salt - Not the Iodized Kind
- Seaweed - Adds a salty flavor to salads
- Raw Nuts and Seeds
- Goji Berries - Great in Smoothies
- Raw Organic Coconut Flakes
- Raw Tahini - Goes in the family of nut and seed butters
- Spices (raw, organic) - Good for adding extra flavor, but don't go overboard
- Herbs
- Spirulina

Some detoxing effects are to be expected, after all your body is purging years of backed up food that's been festering in your intestines. Not a pretty picture, so imagine how much better you'll feel as a result of your healthy diet reboot instead. Common detox side effects include headache, bad breath, body odor, fatigue, irritability, acne, vomiting and diarrhea. These symptoms do pass, and once they've moved on you'll enjoy abundant energy, radiant skin, better sleep, and a clear mind. Enemas, colonic flushing, implants, skin brushing, and moderate exercise will help remove toxins from your system quickly and help the detox process.

Should you experience severe detox symptoms which make it difficult to function normally, ease off the cleansing by adding some raw foods back into your diet and see your physician as soon as possible. Many individuals reported weight loss as a side effect of a raw food cleanse, this is normal. See your doctor before beginning any sort of cleanse, whether short or long term, to establish a baseline measure of your health. This initial checkup will help your doctor monitor the effects of your raw food cleanse to ensure your diet is sufficient.

How to Alkalize Your Body

If you've ever owned a swimming pool, you've probably tested the PH of the water and treated it accordingly to bring it into balance. Something few people realize is the human body requires a PH balance as well. When we're too acidic we experience the side effects in the form of headaches, skin troubles, and excess fat around the abdomen.

Excess acid is stored in fat cells as a means of protecting vital organs, so in some ways it could be said your extra pounds are helpful, but there are easier ways to achieve good health. Begin by drinking the minimum advised amount of water per day. Filtered water is the best, but if you don't have any on hand then distilled water works just as well. In a pinch you can enjoy water straight from the tap with a dash of baking soda tossed in for instant alkalizing effects. To determine the minimum advised amount that's right for you, divide your body weight in half, and drink that amount in ounces each day. Your body may need more or less depending on your environment and how much you sweat, so adjust accordingly.

In addition to drinking enough water each day, make sure you're eating vegetables with high water content, many of which have alkalizing effects on the body as well. Enjoy these as a salad, or blended into a green drink for a quick delivery of natural energizers. The list of which alkalizing foods you can eat freely is rather extensive, so you should never have to worry about diversity or variety in your diet, but if you're unsure of where to begin this list should offer assistance:

- Bell Pepper (Yellow, Orange, or Red)
- Celery
- Cucumber
- Kale
- Lettuce
- Onion
- Romaine
- Spinach
- Wheat Grass
- Zucchini
- Limes
- Lemon

- Tomato
- Avocado
- Olive Oil
- Flax Seed Oil
- Almonds
- Pine Nuts
- Hazelnuts
- Sunflower Seeds

As your body becomes more balance on the PH scale and moves towards greater alkalinity you will notice several positive side effects. Headaches, cravings, and joint pain will disappear, you'll enjoy more restful sleep, and your skin will appear more youthful, clear, and radiant as a result.

Losing Weight with a Raw Food Diet

Losing weight is a normal side effect when following a diet which primarily consists of raw and living foods. This doesn't mean you should take up this diet strictly for the purpose of losing weight. If you're naturally slender and have concerns that this lifestyle will cause you to lose more weight, put your worries aside. Many have found that their weight becomes more stable, and the abundant energy from consuming delicious fruits and vegetables allows them to enjoy an active lifestyle and a healthy appearance.

Much of the weight you can expect to lose will come from years of built up food and waste sitting in your intestines. After all, it takes 3 days to fully digest red meat, compared to 13 hours for vegetables and leafy greens, or 6 hours for fruit. Imagine the sort of gastric traffic jam you've got going on in your intestines if you eat red meat every day!

How to Look Younger Using the Raw Food Diet

Turning back the hands of time is certainly possible, and it doesn't require expensive creams, or lotions, let alone invasive procedures. All it takes is a healthy diet filled with plenty of organic, raw and living foods. Not only will you extend your life, you'll look younger as well.

The secret is not what you put on your skin; it's what you put into your body. Healthy eating is the real fountain of youth! Eating raw fruits, vegetables, greens, seeds and nuts will have you looking younger by your next birthday.

A majority of people who switch to a raw food diet report a more youthful, glowing complexion, while others experience a reduction in wrinkles and others notice a reduction in gray hair. All this from eating a diet of raw and living foods! A simple way to get started is by having a delicious green drink every morning, filled with celery, spinach, cucumber and some apple for sweetness. Savory veggie stews and blended salads are another great way to get more greens into your diet as well.

Boost Your Health with Raw Foods

Your body is able to heal itself naturally, provided you're fueling yourself with the right foods. The problem most of us run into is our unhealthy diet of processed food and animal products actually leads to chronic illness. When your body is struggling to digest meat and processed meals with little-to-no nutritive value, it doesn't have enough energy left to repair the damage done over time by a poor diet.

The good news is this can be easily reversed by following a diet of raw and living foods. Mineral-rich leafy greens are packed with nutrients and vitamins to give your body the fuel it needs, and when blended into a delicious green drink the energy-boosting benefits are practically instantaneous.

Some individuals have been won over to a raw food diet after witnessing miraculous changes in someone they love. It's not a fairy tale that people have cured themselves of cancer, arthritis, asthma, even thyroid issues, as a result of following a diet of raw and living foods.

Nutritional Benefits of Raw Food Diet

One of the first things people notice when they begin a raw food diet is a significant increase in their energy levels. Some even take up exercise and physically demanding hobbies to take advantage of this abundance of energy. You'll also find you have plenty of extra time as well, since you won't be spending so much time preparing your meals.

In addition to increased energy, you'll also experience more restful sleep. When you happen to feel like sleeping that is because some people report less need for sleep as a result of feeling so super-charged. Peaceful sleep and the sensation of blissful relaxation which accompanies a raw food diet will also improve the appearance of your skin.

After just one week of eating raw foods, you'll notice a healthy glow to your skin, clearer eyes, and a reduction of wrinkles. People will think you've had a facelift, just imagine their surprise when you explain the secret is simply enjoying what nature provides.

Should all this fail to be convincing, you'll also notice a decrease in chronic conditions such as heart disease, diabetes and cancer. Your doctor will also be able to measure a significant reduction in cholesterol and triglyceride levels. Your thyroid will also function better, and you'll experience fewer digestion complaints.

Naturally you'll want to consult your doctor before starting any sort of drastic change in diet or routine. This will help establish a baseline measurement of your health so you can track your progress on multiple levels, as well as make any corrections as needed should any deficiencies occur. When deficiencies do occur it's generally because there aren't enough leafy greens in the diet. Juicing is the easiest method by far to ensure enough leafy greens are consumed each day.

Chapter 5: TECHNIQUES IN PREPARING RAW

Cutting and Chopping Techniques

Even though you won't be doing any traditional cooking, you're still going to prep some food every once in a while. Because you'll want to impress your friends with your delicious new recipes, you'll probably want to polish your cutting and chopping skills as well.

Always begin with a cutting board and flat, sturdy surface to work on. There's nothing worse than trying to cut something in half while fighting against an uneven surface. Give yourself plenty of room to work on as well. A cramped work surface is a stressful work surface. When cutting round items it's easiest to slice off a small section off one end, leaving you with a flat surface that will keep your food from trying to escape.

The different techniques described here will be useful for any number of recipes, so you can always enjoy interesting and diverse meals from one day to the next. Some juicers claim to allow easy processing of whole fruits and vegetables, and for the most part it's true. To extend the life of your juicer, however, it's a good idea to break down some of the more fibrous plants into pieces, such as celery.

Chopping – Chopping, in essence, is cutting food into small, manageable pieces. When chopping it's best to use a knife that is twice the size of what you're cutting, this will allow for easier leverage and less strain for you.

Grip the knife handle firmly while pinching the blade between your thumb and forefinger, this will allow for greater control over the knife while cutting. Always keep the point of the knife in contact with your cutting board to ensure yet another level of control over the blade.

With your other hand, grip your fruit, vegetable, or greens, firmly, with your fingertips curled under slightly, well out of the way of the blade. Leverage your blade in smooth strokes. You should be able to maintain contact with the cutting board without much trouble. The trick is to move the food, not the knife. The blade of your knife need only move up and down while you carefully push the food along for even slices. Chop as large or as small as you wish, but try for uniform pieces as a way to improve your technique.

Mincing - Mincing follows the same technique as chopping. The goal is simply to achieve extra small pieces. Onions, garlic, and shallots are most often served minced. Mincing doesn't require pretty, perfect little pieces, so it's okay to go a little knife-happy so long as your fingers are well out of the way.

Dicing - Dicing is just like chopping, but usually with more steps in order to achieve small, cube-shaped pieces. Anything can be diced, even carrots and potatoes. Simply chop into slices, cut these slices into sticks, then cut once more into cubes. Dicing does take some practice, but it's quite easy to do once you get the hang of it.

What is Juicing?

Did you know it takes three days to digest red meat? Compare that to the 9-12 hours it takes to digest fruits and vegetables, and the impressive 6 hours it takes to fully digest juice and it becomes a little more apparent why so many people are carrying around excess fat. They're still digesting a meal from three days ago!

Juice cleanses are often recommended to individuals who wish to reverse the damaging effects from a lifetime of poor eating habits. Juicing is recommended not only because it's easier to digest, allowing the body greater time to start the healing process, but also because the body starts metabolizing juice instantly. Meaning you'll feel the energizing effects within fifteen minutes of drinking a green juice.

Juicing is also packed with vital nutrients. Plus it's just easier. Imagine eating a pound of crunchy carrots. Now imagine drinking that pound of juicy carrots. Starting each day with a green drink consisting of spinach, cucumber, kale, lemon, and apple will leave you feeling instantly energized.

Juicing does require special equipment in the form of a juicer. It's a good idea to visit a shop and asks questions to determine which model is the best for your particular needs. Some juicers are made specifically for citrus fruits, allowing you to simply slice the fruit in half and extract the fruit, while others allow you to feed in whole pieces of fruit without any trouble.

Dehydration and Raw Food

Dehydrated food can last up to a few months so long as all the water is removed. Store your food in an airtight container, at room temperature or in the refrigerator. Or store it in a glass container, if you can, to maintain an airtight seal for greater longevity.

If you're in a humid environment, store your dehydrated food in the refrigerator. Otherwise the food will pull any available moisture from the air.

Rather than worry about temperature settings, simply keep the heat set at 105 degrees.

I like to experiment with what I dehydrate; it's kind of like a science experiment. When I first started a raw food diet, I was dreadful at making smoothies. My problem was I always wanted something complicated, filled with several different ingredients. This works great with juices, but for some reason it just didn't work with my early smoothies.

Not one to throw in the towel, I'd pour these sad smoothies onto a dehydrator pan, transforming them into a delicious tropical fruit leather. These worked great as wraps too, and as fruit leather, a real happy accident. The point is, experiment and play around, you'll be surprised how many things you can dehydrate.

How to Do Blanching and Steaming?

Transitioning to a raw food diet can be difficult for some, but there are a few things you can do to make your cooked food a little better for you. Blanching and steaming are two ways of quick cooking your food which preserve the most nutritive value. As with any cooking method nutritive value is lost once heat is applied to your food.

Raw food purists believe that nothing you eat should be cooked, but in the case of broccoli and asparagus a quick blanching makes the food easier to digest. It all comes down to personal preference, and your body's needs, if you must have cooked food at least try it steamed or blanched so it's as close to raw as possible.

To blanch your food, drop it into boiling water and boil for 2-6 minutes depending on the type of food. Corn needs a longer blanch time; asparagus needs less time. Remove the food from the boiling water and immediately drop into an ice bath to stop the cooking process. Blanching corn in this manner will keep it fresh for storage.

In the case of steaming, your food comes into contact with far less water compared to blanching. Blanching works best for some things, while steaming works best for others. When steaming broccoli, add a small amount of water to your cooking pot, usually enough water to cover the bottom of the pot followed by some handfuls of broccoli florets. Bring water to a boil and cook, covered, for 3 minutes. Your broccoli should be crisp yet tender, top with some tamari for a delicious side dish.

What Is Sprouting?

Just as nuts have protective enzyme inhibitors which keep them dormant in their raw state, the same is true for seeds. Sprouted seeds are packed with nutrients, they are living plants supercharged with enzymes. You don't need to have a green thumb to successfully sprout seeds; you just need a clean, well-ventilated place to allow them to do what they're made to do.

Some seeds you can enjoy almost immediately, others need a few days to grow, the process of sprouting remains the same for each. Start by soaking your seeds. Overnight tends to be the common amount of time for the majority of seeds and nuts, with a few exceptions to the rule here and there to keep things interesting.

After a good soaking, drain well, and evenly distribute within your chosen sprouting container. Glass jars can be used for sprouting, or specially made bags which retain moisture. There are even special sprouting machines available, experiment to find the container that's best for you.

Allow your container to drain thoroughly, but don't let your seeds get too dry. Rinse and drain your sprouts two or three times each day, taking time to give your sprouting container a gentle shake to distribute your sprouts again. This allows for better draining and room for your sprouts to grow. After a day or so you'll see little tails sprouting from your seeds. In another day or two you'll be able to remove the hulls.

Removing the hulls is a personal preference. Your sprouts shed the hulls of their original seed naturally. If you would like to remove the hulls of your sprouts, fill a large bowl with water and place your sprouts into the bowl. The hulls will float to the top which you can then skim off with a spoon. Return your sprouts to their container and allow them to grow a little more. Once they're grown to your liking, allow them to dry completely and store in an airtight container for up to a week.

Chapter 6: SAMPLE RAW RECIPES AND TIPS

How to Make Raw Food Smoothies

A green smoothie is basically fruits and greens blended with some water. There's no real rule or science to the amount of fruits to add versus greens, so you're free to experiment with local fruits and produce. If you don't like dark leafy greens, add celery instead so you can still get nutrition and fiber. If you're having trouble finding seasonal fruit, frozen fruit will work in a pinch.

The goal is to blend up a smoothie that isn't lumpy, isn't going to separate, or suffering from a foam of chlorophyll at the top which isn't difficult once you understand the difference between the two types of fiber present in your fruits and greens. Basically it comes down to soluble fibers and insoluble fibers. For reference, insolvable fibers are the kinds we weave fabrics and materials from. Greens are a good source of insoluble fiber which is good for removing toxins and waste from the body.

To make a good smoothie that's creamy and satisfying you need a plentiful source of soluble fiber to blend with the insoluble fiber. This will not only result in a creamier, more satisfying smoothie, it will also taste naturally sweet. Great sources of soluble fiber include:

- Bananas
- Pears
- Kiwi
- Strawberry
- Papaya
- Peaches

Mangos are a fiber superfruit, containing both soluble and insoluble fiber. Keep it simple at first, one or two fruits along with some greens, and experiment with more complex blends. Toss in some superfood like hemp seeds and goji berries for an extra kick. Remember to chew your smoothie to activate the process of digestion.

Tropical Smoothie
- Banana
- Mango

- Pear
- Strawberries
- Apples
- Spinach
- Water

Morning Energizer
- Banana - one
- Hemp Seeds - tbsp
- Dulse - pinch
- Blueberries – ½ cup
- Kale - greens removed from the spine, about a cup worth

Fruit Smoothie
- Orange
- Banana
- Frozen blueberries
- Coconut water or Water
- Greens, Cup of Kale, Celery, Romaine Lettuce, Collards

Potassium Powerhouse
- Coconut water (two coconuts)
- Figs (two)
- Bananas (five)
- Head of Kale

Farmer's Market Smoothie
- Half Pear
- Banana
- Cup of Frozen Mango
- Flaxseed
- 1 or 2 medjool dates.

The savory green smoothie is a nice change of pace when you're in the mood for something satisfying, but not sweet. Add the tomatoes to the blender first, followed by the spinach and parsley. The water content in the tomatoes will help blend the greens better. Next, break up the celery into chunks to make their tough fibers easier to process for the blender. Add your remaining ingredients, throwing in just enough hot pepper to suit your taste. Or leave it out completely if you don't want the extra zing of heat in your smoothie. Blend to a smooth consistency, pour into a glass and serve.

Savory Green Smoothie
- Spinach
- Celery
- Spicy Pepper
- Avocado
- Tomato
- Parsley

Blended Salad Smoothie
- Oranges
- Cucumber
- Chia seeds
- Banana
- Avocado
- Ginger
- Romaine lettuce
- Cherry tomatoes

How to Make Raw Food Bars

Raw food bars are a great way to combine the nutritious benefits of fruits and nuts with the satisfying texture of a protein bar. If you're looking for something chewy, filling and packed with nutrients then a bar is the treat for you. Each of these recipes will keep for about a week if stored in an airtight container in the refrigerator.

Almond Indulgence Bar
1 cup Raw Almond Butter
1 cup Coconut Oil
¼ cup Sprouted/dehydrated Buckwheat
1/3 cup Goji Berries
1/3 cup Lucuma Powder

Almond butter and coconut oil, equal parts into a food processor. Add in a bit of Lucuma powder for sweetness, blend on high until you've reached a liquid consistency. Add buckwheat and goji berries, then pulse to blend. Spoon into small containers and place in freezer to desired firmness, about five minutes.

Zesty Lemon Bars

1 cup soaked almonds
2 pitted Madjool Dates
Zest of one lemon
Squeeze of lemon

Blend to a sticky, crumbly consistency. Place some wax paper into a dish, then spread almond and date paste into dish, forming a solid bar. Shape into an even thickness, and then cut into smaller bars for easy serving. Place in freezer for about an hour to firm up before serving.

Truly Raw Chocolate Bars

1 cup pitted organic Dates
1 cup sun dried raisins
1 cup soaked almonds
½ cup hemp seeds
¼ cup raw cacao powder
4 tablespoons organic coconut oil
¼ cup raw cacao nibs
½ cup goji berries
Pinch of Dulse

Spread coconut oil into a glass dish to keep bars from sticking. Blend ingredients in a food processor until crumbly and sticky. Consistency is really a matter of preference; some like a thick paste others like more texture. Spread into a pan, cover and refrigerate until firm. Slice into bars and serve.

Coconutty Lemon Bars

1 cup soaked almonds
1 ½ cups pitted medjool dates.
Seeds of 1 vanilla been
Pinch of dulse
Zest of one lemon
2 tablespoons lemon juice
1 cup shredded, dried coconut meat.

Process the almonds in a food processor into small pieces. Use a bit of the powdered almond to dust the bottom of a square pan. Add remaining ingredients and process until blended well. Spread into dish and press to distribute evenly. Chill until firm, about two hours, and cut into squares.

How to Make Raw Food Desserts

Raw deserts taste great, and they're good for you as well, because they're free of refined sugars, processed flour and unhealthy fats. Raw desserts are also easy to make and oftentimes take just a few minutes to prepare. Just about any dessert can be made into a raw food variant with just a few simple substitutions. Round nuts and coconut take the place of flour and butter, dried fruits replace sweeteners, and avocado replaces cream, butter and eggs. Usually you want soaked nuts for recipes, but not necessarily in the case of pie crusts where you want something more crumbly and dry in consistency.

Chocolate Pudding Pie
Crust:
½ cup walnuts
½ cup pecans
1 cup shredded coconut
Pinch of salt
4-6 medjool dates

Filling:
Soaked dates
Agave Nectar
Vanilla Extract
2 Mashed avocadoes
Splash of water
1 cup Organic Cocoa powder or raw cocoa powder

Blend nuts, coconut and salt in food processor until resembling coarse crumbs. Add dates and blend until the mixture is sticky and pliable like dough. Evenly distribute crust into a pie plate and press firmly into place. Place crust in refrigerator while preparing filling. Blend dates, vanilla and agave nectar in food processor then add avocado, followed by cocoa powder, blending thoroughly after each. Add water if necessary to achieve a smooth consistency. Spoon into pie plate and spread evenly. Refrigerate for two hours before serving.

Coconut Date Roll
2 cups pitted dates
1 cup raisins
Grated coconut
1 cup chopped pecans or almonds

Grind dates and raisins in a food processor till sticky and crumbly, mix
in nuts by hand. Using a teaspoon for measuring, roll date and nut
paste into small, even balls, and then roll in shredded coconut to coat.

Chia Seed Pudding
2 ½ cups almond milk
3 tablespoons agave nectar
½ cup chia seeds
½ tsp lemon zest, finely grated

In a one quart jar, combine almond milk with the agave nectar. Close
the jar and shake vigorously to combine. Add remaining ingredients to
the jar close once more and shake well again. Refrigerate till desired
consistency, generally 4 hours to overnight. Shake or stir occasionally,
and serve in individual bowls

Chocolate Banana Tart
Crust:
1 cup Shredded Coconut
1 cup Almonds
¼ tsp cayenne
½ tsp celtic sea salt
1 cup Barhi Dates, chopped

Filling:
1 Avocado
½ cup cacao
1 tablespoon gluten free vanilla
½ cup agave nectar

Blend coconut, almonds, cayenne and sea salt in a food processor to a
crumbly consistency, and then add barhi dates to make the mixture
sticky. If the crust is not as sticky as you'd like, add a bit of agave
nectar. Blend ingredients for filling in food processor till smooth,

spread half in pie plate, top with sliced banana, cover with remaining chocolate mousse.

Chocolate Blueberry Pie
Basic Crust:
1 ¼ c Almonds, soaked
6 Dates, soaked
Dash of cinnamon
1 tsp vanilla
Water as needed for moisture

Filling:
2 cups blueberries
2 cups cashews
2 tablespoons raw cacao powder
2 tablespoons agave nectar

Grind to a fine, crumbly texture. Press into a pie plate, starting in the middle and working carefully towards the edges. Let the crust hang out in the refrigerator for an hour or two to firm up before making filling. Blend all filling ingredients in a food processor or blender, spoon filling into pie crust and smooth evenly. Place in the freezer for at least one hour before serving, and allow to thaw about 10 minutes for easier slicing.

Cheesecake with Strawberries
Crust:
2 cups soaked nuts (blend of almonds, walnuts and pecans)
½ cup soaked, pitted dates
2 chopped carrots
1 tablespoon cinnamon

Cheese:
1 cup soaked cashews
1 cup soaked, pitted dates
1 ½ cup strawberries
1 tablespoon vanilla
Agar agar soaked in a half cup of warm water for 30 minutes
½ cup water
Stevia to taste

Blend crust ingredients in a food processor until crumbly and a little sticky. Press into a pan to create the bottom crust of the cheesecake. Blend filling ingredients in a food processor until fluffy and light, and sweeten as necessary to suit your taste. Spread over crust, and then place in refrigerator for at least three hours to firm up.

Coconut Ice Cream
½ cup water
¼ cup soaked cashews
¼ cup macadamia nuts
¼ cup coconut butter
3 tablespoons coconut sugar
Squeeze of lime juice
1 tsp cacao nibs
Pinch of dulse
Stevia to taste

Blend all ingredients in a food processor or a high-powered blender. Other fruits can be added for extra sweetness, this is a basic recipe that goes well with banana, mango and other fruit. Pour into a bowl and place in the freezer, stirring every 30 minutes until the consistency of ice cream.

How to Make Raw Food Bacon

Food cravings are bound to occur when you begin transitioning to a raw food diet. Most often, when those cravings strikes, the food of choice is something savory, salty, and comforting, compared to something sugary. The craving which derails most raw foodists is for bacon.

The thing to consider here isn't so much the bacon itself that's the object of craving, but more of the savory, salty, crispy satisfaction of the sweet and smoky treat. Since this is what the body is really craving, it's easy to deliver without going off your diet.

This brings us to the subject of raw bacon. Yes it really exists, and it's actually good for you! Eggplant or aubergines depending on your location, tend to be the vegetable of choice for the base of the recipe, but zucchini, summer squash, shitake mushrooms, and thinly sliced jicima work just as well. Coconut is another satisfying substitution for raw bacon.

The process for all of these recipes is exactly the same, regardless of the type of base vegetable you're using. Marinate for two hours and then dehydrate overnight at 110 degrees. Turn halfway through dehydrating for an even crispness. Check as often as needed to achieve desired crispness. As an added bonus, these marinades can be used as salad dressings as well.

Here you will find three variations of basic marinade to use for eggplants, zucchini, squash and jicima. Feel free to experiment with flavors that are satisfying to your taste. Two additional recipes are included for coconut and shitake bacon should you wish to try something with a meatier texture.

Marinade One
2 tbsp tamari / nama shoyu
2 tbsp Agave nectar
2 tbsp apple cider vinegar
2 tbsp olive oil
1 tsp cumin
1 tsp chili powder
3-5 drops liquid smoke
2 cloves of garlic, minced
Black pepper to taste

Marinade Two
¾ cup Olive Oil
2 tbsp Raw Honey
4 tbsp Ume Plum Vinegar
Cayenne Pepper to taste

Marinade Three
¼ cup Teriyaki Sauce
¼ cup Hemp Oil
Juice from half a lemon
Red pepper flakes
1 tsp raw sugar
½ tsp celtic sea salt
Minced dulse, one strip or two
1 clove grated garlic
1 tbsp smoked paprika

Coconut Bacon
Meat from 2 coconuts
¾ cup macadamia nuts
¼ cup coconut oil
½ cup coconut water
¼ cup tamari
Salt and Pepper to taste

Shitake Bacon
8 ounces Shitake mushrooms, sliced*
¼ cup Tamari
¼ cup Braggs liquid aminos
Splash of olive oil
*stems can be used if they're not too woody

How to Make Raw Food Spaghetti

Pasta is a comforting main dish which most people avoid because of the high carbohydrate and starch content. When people crave pasta, what they really are looking for is that al dente texture paired with a rich, flavorful sauce. Pasta on its own doesn't have a whole lot of flavor; it's pretty much a carrier for the sauce.

Zucchini is also bland on its own, and has a nice firm texture, making it an ideal substitute for pasta when sliced properly. One to two zucchinis is perfect per person, and spiral slicers make preparation a breeze. You can also use a food processor or a vegetable peeler if you'd like to experiment with different textures.

The most basic raw spaghetti recipes consist of three ingredients only: zucchini, tomatoes and basil. When sliced with a vegetable peeler, your zucchini will have a texture and appearance similar to fettuccini. Simply peel around the vegetable until you get to the core. Set the core aside for a delicious garden vegetable soup. When choosing zucchini for raw pasta, you should look for a one that isn't too old and has a nice thick diameter.

Spiral slicers can also be used and the result is much more like angel hair pasta. Cut the zucchini to fit into the spiral slicer, you may need to cut your zucchini down to sections of two or three pieces. Set zucchini firmly in place within the spiral slicer, and crank away to create long strands of vegetable pasta.

Though you can use a blender for your marinara sauce, it's recommended that you use a food processor instead because this will maintain some texture and chunkiness to the final product. You can warm up your sauce slightly; no one ever said that raw food had to be cold food. Stir constantly while warming up your sauce and don't warm it any higher than body temperature.

Basic Spaghetti
Zucchini, sliced to your preference
Tomatoes
Bunch of Basil
Blend tomato and basil together in a blender till smooth, toss with zucchini and serve.

Satisfying and Savory Spaghetti
2 cups tomato, sliced
1 red bell pepper
½ cup sun-dried tomatoes
1 garlic clove, minced
Pinch of salt, to taste
1/8 cup olive oil
Pinch of Cayenne
Black pepper to taste.

If your sun-dried tomatoes are especially dry, soak them for about 20 minutes before adding to the food processor. Sun-dried tomatoes make an excellent thickener and have a wonderfully sweet tomato taste. Blend all ingredients in a food processor till well blended, scraping down the sides as needed.

Prepare zucchini as desired, using either a vegetable peeler, spiral slicer or food processor. Toss marinara zucchini a few minutes before serving. Sauce can be served warm or cold, and will keep in the refrigerator for up to a week.

Spaghetti Squash with Pesto:
1 bunch fresh basil leaves
1 cup soaked walnuts

5 cloves fresh garlic
1 teaspoon sea salt
1/3 cup olive oil
1 Spaghetti Squash, sliced thin

Process everything but the squash in a food processor till well blended. Peel the skin from the squash using a vegetable peeler then slice with a mandolin, or spiral slicer. Top squash with pesto and serve.

How to Plan Raw Food Menus

Planning your menu from one day to the next is actually quite simple and takes very little effort. In the case of dehydrated foods some planning ahead is necessary, but much of these menu items keep for a good while so you won't constantly be preparing something today for you to enjoy tomorrow.

Flax Crackers, sprouted bread, and other dehydrated foods can be prepared on a weekend afternoon for you to enjoy throughout the entire week. Should you desire something comforting for breakfast, such as oatmeal, simply purchase sprouting oats and soak them overnight in your blender with some water and cinnamon, add in some apple slices in the morning then blend until combined.

Milk for homemade cereal can be easily blended from nuts that have soaked for 24-48 hours. Simply place soaked nuts into a blender with 2 cups of water, blend until smooth then strain through a cheese cloth. Squeeze the cheesecloth firmly to drain as much liquid as possible, return the nut paste within the cheese cloth to the blender and repeat as often as you wish.

Keep this nut paste though, it makes a fabulous base for spreads and butters; simply add herbs or sweeten to taste. A sample menu is provided, along with alternatives, but this just barely scratches the surface of all the options available to you on a raw food diet. For more suggestions and ideas, simply browse the internet until you find a raw recipe that sounds appealing and give it a try!

Day One:
Breakfast -

Green Smoothie made with banana, apple, orange, huge handful of spinach or kale, splash of lemon, and a dash of cinnamon.
OR
Raw Oatmeal made with sproutable oats, water, apple and cinnamon.
OR
Cereal made with crisp apple slices, chopped soaked almonds, a dash of cinnamon and a drizzle of honey. Top with soaked flax seeds and cashew milk.

Snack -
Fruit Smoothie

Lunch -
Big salad with a small amount of fat such as a dressing made with avocado, tomato, flax seeds and a drizzle of olive oil. The secret to this salad is to really mix it well, making sure to incorporate all of the ingredients.

Snack -
Fruit
OR
Handful of soaked nuts
OR
Carrot sticks

Dinner -
Raw flaxseed crackers
Savory nut pate
Sliced vegetables

Desert -
Chia pudding

Works Cited

40 Year Medical Doctor on Benefits of Raw Foods and Water Fasting. Life Regenerator. March 2011. August 2012. *http://www.youtube.com/watch?v=OgcwvpGzeSQ*

6 Tips to Stay on a Raw Food Diet. The Raw Food Family. July 2012. July 2012. *http://www.youtube.com/watch?v=jyS0l14pClg*

7 Biggest Mistakes on a Raw Food Diet. The Raw Food Family. May 2009.

July 2012. *http://www.youtube.com/watch?v=HjCrtKmFshI*

70 Year Old Woman Looks Young – Raw Foods Diet. Lawrence Jay. July 2012. July 2012. *http://www.youtube.com/watch?v=ADzAJUsSZn0*

Alkaline Foods* Acid Alkaline Diet* Alkalize Your Body. Life Regenerator. August 2009. August 2012. *http://www.youtube.com/watch?v=Nhlj0hjes7w*

Alkalize Your Body for Great Digestion, Immunity and Overall Health. Rachel's Wellness. July 2011. August 2012. *http://www.youtube.com/watch?v=cez0mr-AQQ0*

Fat, Sick, and Nearly Dead. Dir. Joe Cross and Kurt Engfehr. Reboot Media

Forks Over Knives. Dir. Lee Fulkerson. Monica Beach Media

How to Chop Vegetables Very Quickly. WikiHow. June 2012. August 2012. *http://www.wikihow.com/Chop-Vegetables-Very-Quickly*

How to Grow Sprouts. Kristens Raw. July 2009. July 2012. *http://www.youtube.com/watch?v=-gkUokxEPeg*

How to Sprout Brown Rice. The Coconut Momma. October 2012. July 2012. *http://www.youtube.com/watch?v=47yjT6whN9A*

How to Start a Raw Food Diet. September, 2009. July 2012. *http://www.youtube.com/watch?v=VFdHRS-aLxU*

No Fat Spaghetti ~ Weight Loss Recipes ~ Raw Vegan Lifestyle. Life Regenerator. October 2011. July *2011.* *http://www.youtube.com/watch?v=ceueqNqvAVQ*

Planning Meals for a Raw Food Diet. The Durian King. January 2012. August 2012. *http://www.youtube.com/watch?v=Q0sRhl2BUh8*

Raw Food Almond Dream Bar. *Raw Reform.* October 2008. August 2012. *http://www.youtube.com/watch?v=XvUiFxlJWLE*

Raw Food Breakfast: Fruit Smoothies and Green Smoothies. Jennifer Cornbleet. September 2009. July 2012. *http://www.youtube.com/watch?v=-G6i9RzyLYk*

RAW FOOD DIET TIPS: Fruit Ripening and Storage. Raw Food Results. November 2011. July 2012.

http://www.youtube.com/watch?v=MY_xqI11CbY

Raw Food Diet Tips: How to Stop Craving Sugary Foods. Ehow Fitness. July 2010. August 2012. *http://www.youtube.com/watch?v=oEiVF5fx_Iw*

Raw Food Diet Too Expensive? How Raw Foods Will Save You Money. OK Raw. March 2012. July 2012. *http://www.youtube.com/watch?v=SYLpCOn3iqM*

Raw Food Recipe: Eggplant Bacon. Living the Raw Life. February 2012. August 2012. *http://www.youtube.com/watch?v=F5wTDdNHaT4*

Raw Food Recipe: Lauren's Lemon Zest Bars #302. Kevin Gianni. May 2009. August 2012. *http://www.youtube.com/watch?v=iQ4izgxFvGk*

Supercharge Me. Dir. Jenna Norwood. Emporia Pictures

Tips for Making & Storing Dehydrated Raw Food, Ep215. Raw Radiant Health. April 2010. July 2012. *http://www.youtube.com/watch?v=j6P0hDTnmr4*

Video 3 – Raw Food Cleanse vs. Other Cleanses. Delicious Revolution. December 2010. August 2012 *http://www.youtube.com/watch?v=B_Y3m1IgCdU*

Zucchini Pasta with Marinara Sauce – A Healthy and Delicious Raw Food Recipe. Jennifer Cornbleet. September 2009. August 2012. *http://www.youtube.com/watch?v=owpk18SyBJg*

www.ingramcontent.com/pod-product-compliance
Lightning Source LLC
Chambersburg PA
CBHW070235290526
45789CB00004B/1634